Why Is My Sugar So Sweet

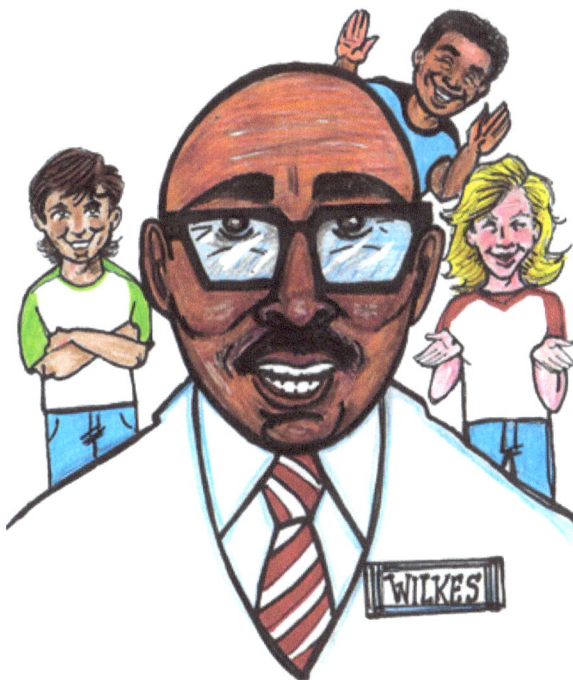

by
Leslie Wilkes

WLL Enterprises, Inc.
An Accredited Business with the Better Business Bureau
P.O. Box 5273, Carson, CA. 90749 USA
www.wllenterprisesinc.org

Copyright 2016, Leslie Wilkes, All Rights Reserved
Book: Why Is My Sugar So Sweet
Date Published: 10/2016 /Edition 1 Trade Paperback
ISBN: 978-0-692-78141-8

This book was published in Compton, California
United States of America

A Publisher Trademark Title Page

WHY IS MY SUGAR SO SWEET

100% of the proceeds from the sale of this book will go to
WLL Enterprises Inc.
WLL Enterprises Inc. is a Non-Profit Organization dedicated
to fighting Childhood Obesity.

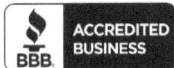

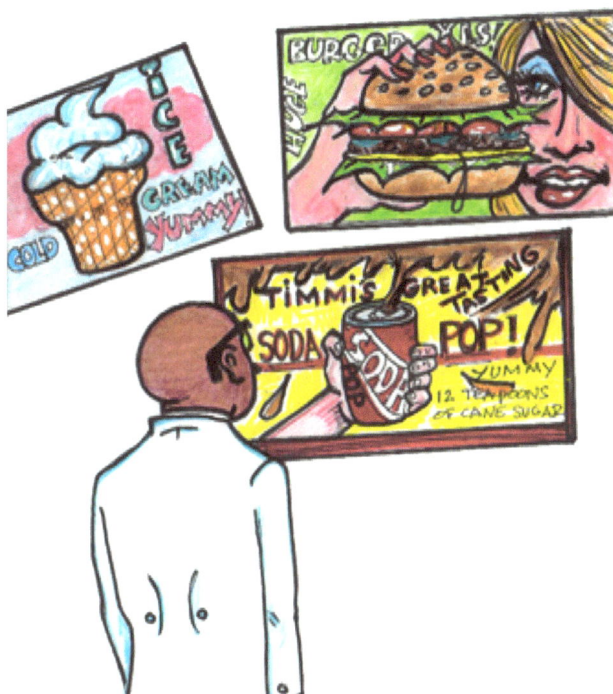

As I walk around and look at billboards and Commercials on TV.....

3

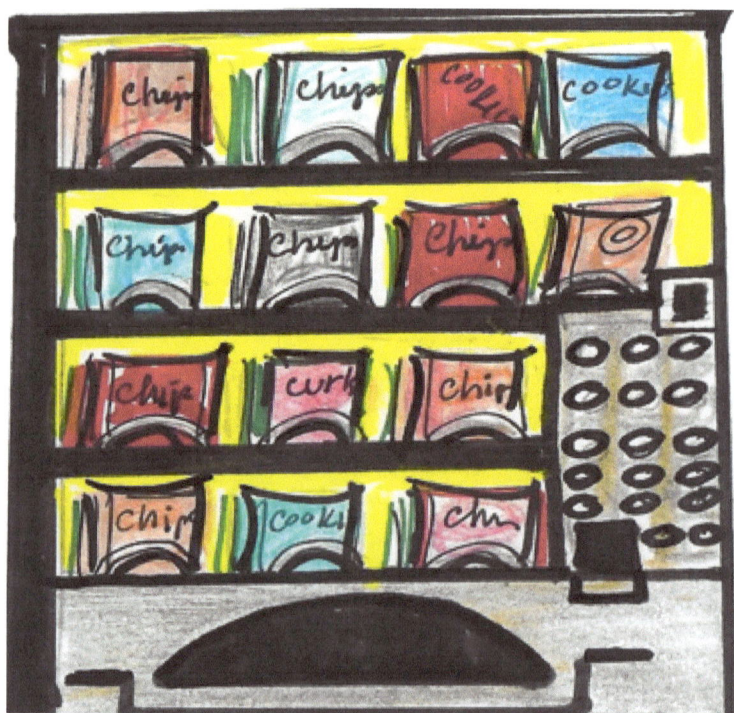

All I see is unhealthy snacks, food and drinks. These are all full of unhealthy choices; chips, candy and sodas.

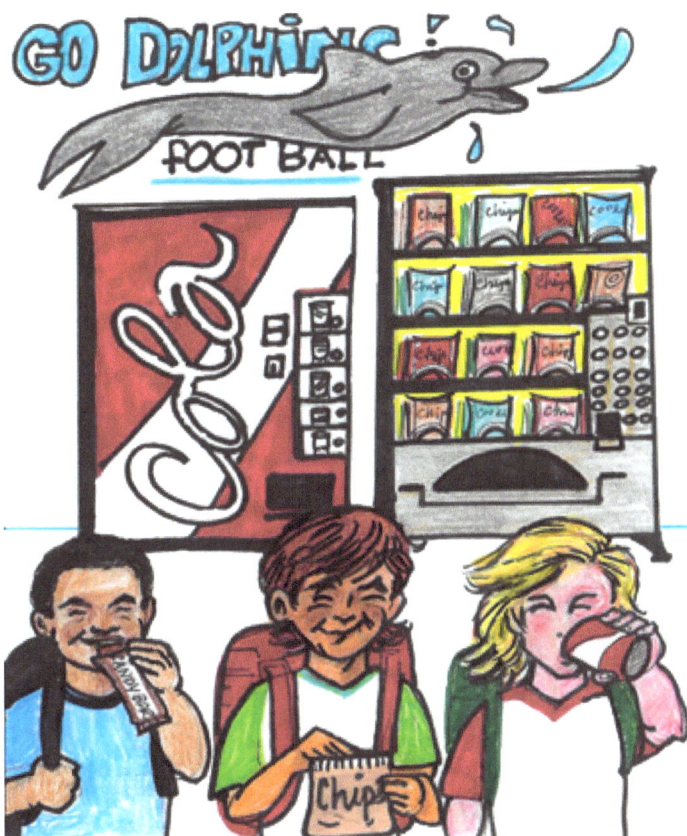

Vending machines in schools....

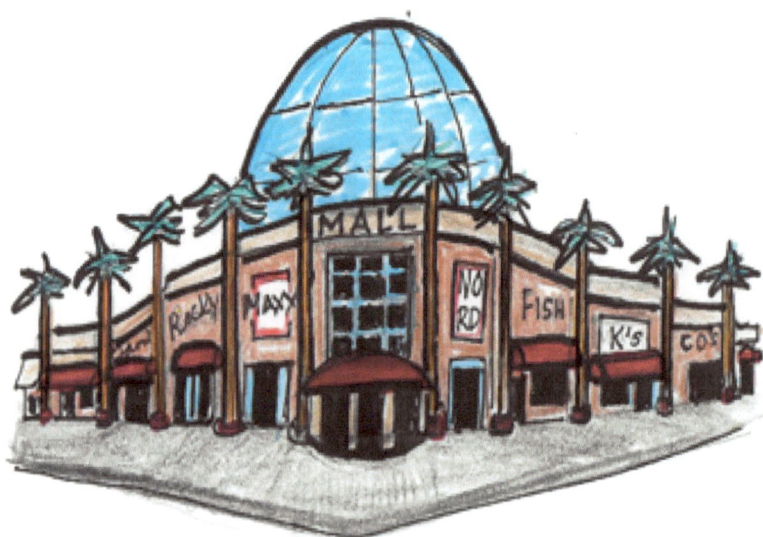

Malls and Shopping centers......

6

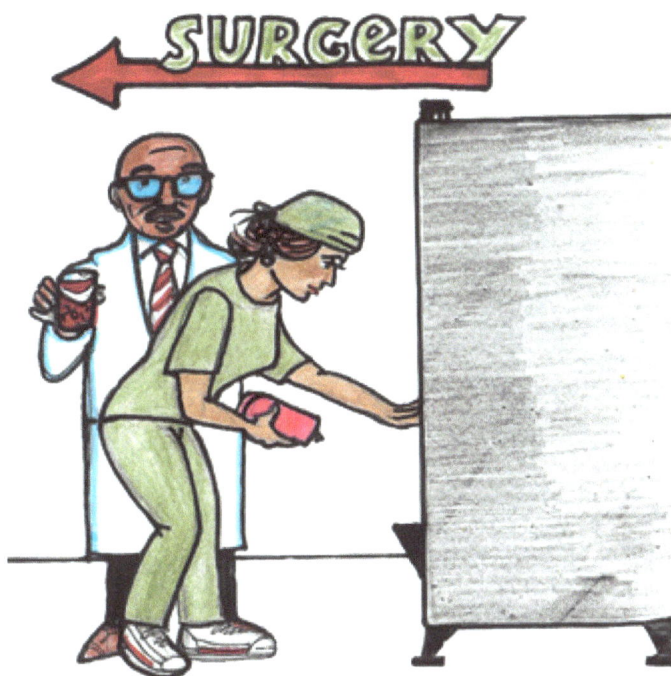

And even hospitals have them.

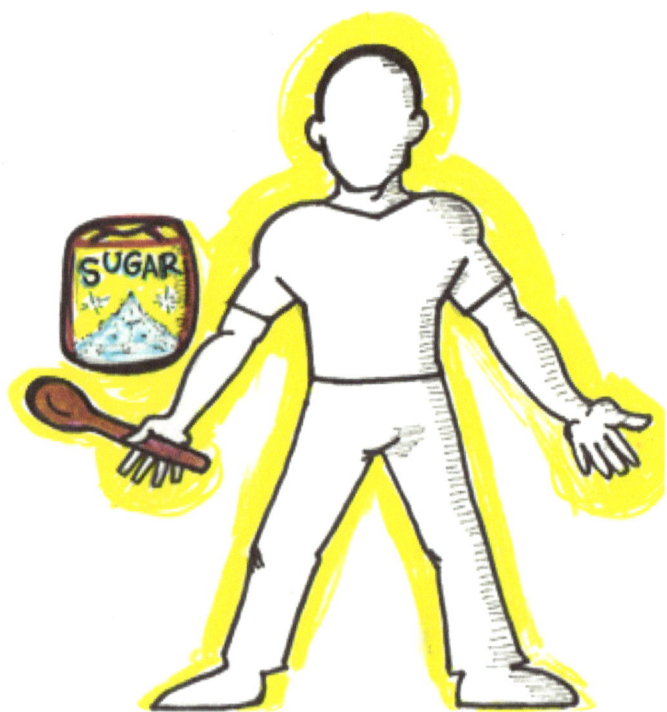

How much sugar does my body need each day?

It is recommended that your body has **NO MORE** than 5 teaspoons of sugar if you're between the ages of 4-6, 6 teaspoons ages 7-10 and 7 teaspoons age 11 years and up.

How do sodas and other drinks measure up?

**You might as well eat
a handful of sugar!**

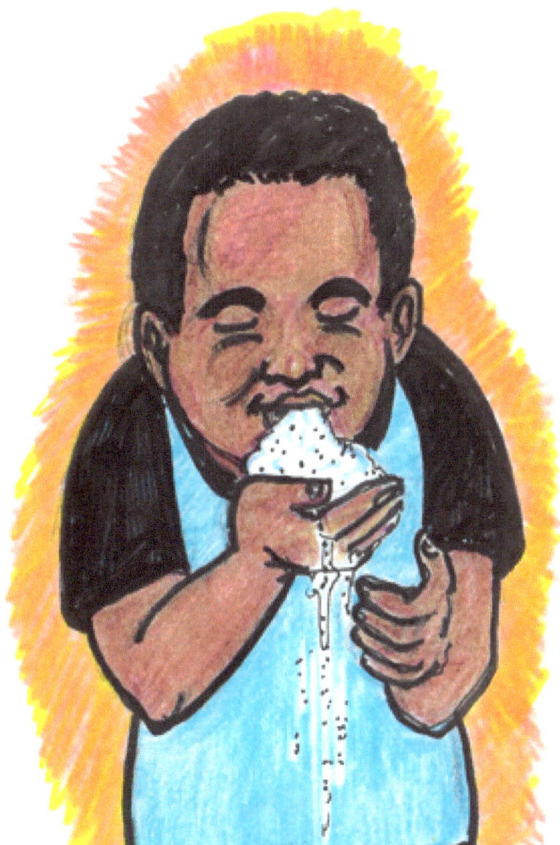

Sodas range from 8 to almost 11 teaspoons of sugar per 12 ounces can.

Energy drinks range from 6 to 7 teaspoons of sugar per 8 ounce serving.

8 ounces of teas, juices and lemonades range from 3 to 6 teaspoons of sugar per serving.

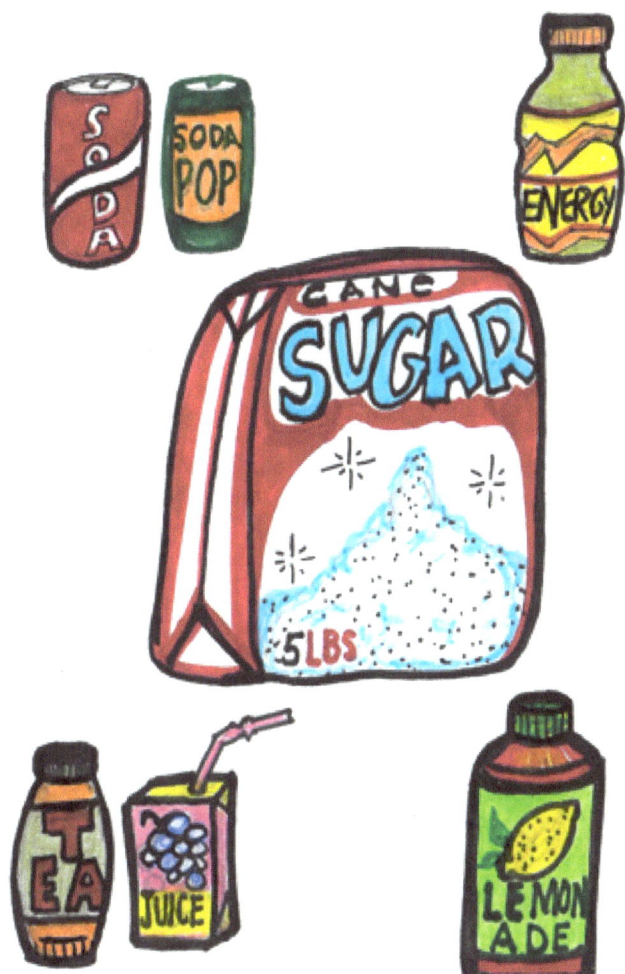

**What effects will that amount
of sugar have on your body?**

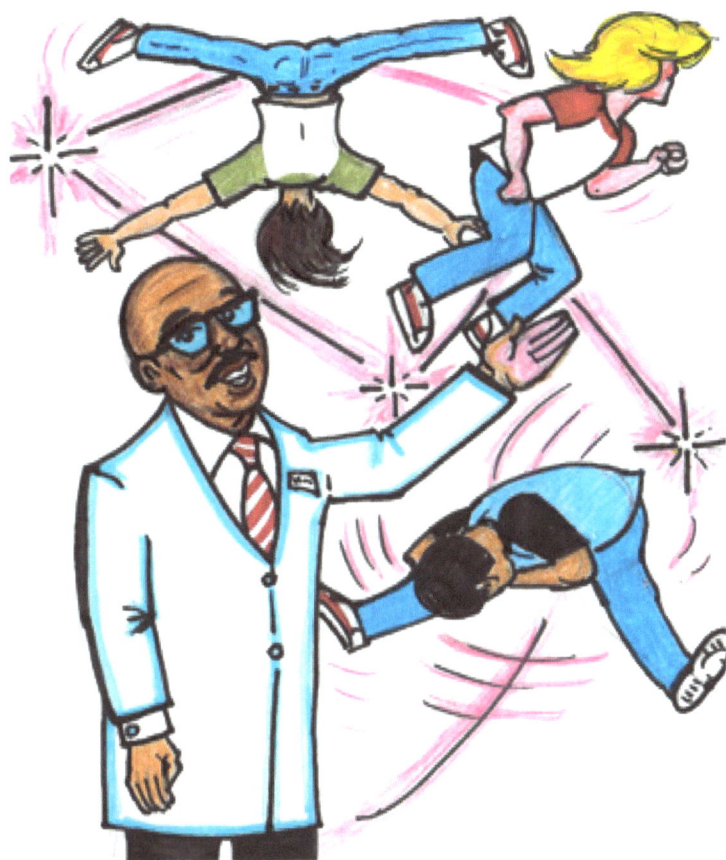

Some parents think it only makes kids bounce off the walls!!

It's worse than that!

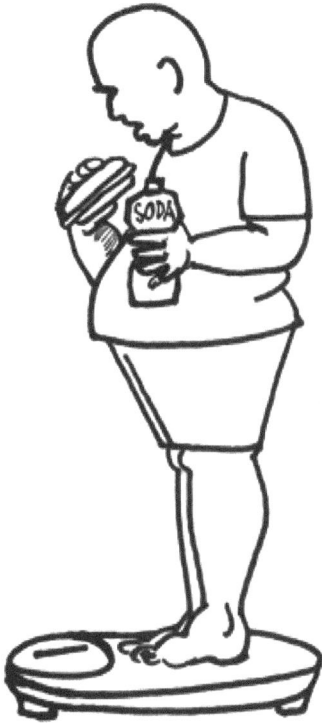

**High intake of sugary foods and drinks
is associated with weight gain that
leads to obesity.**

Obesity leads to diabetes and heart disease.

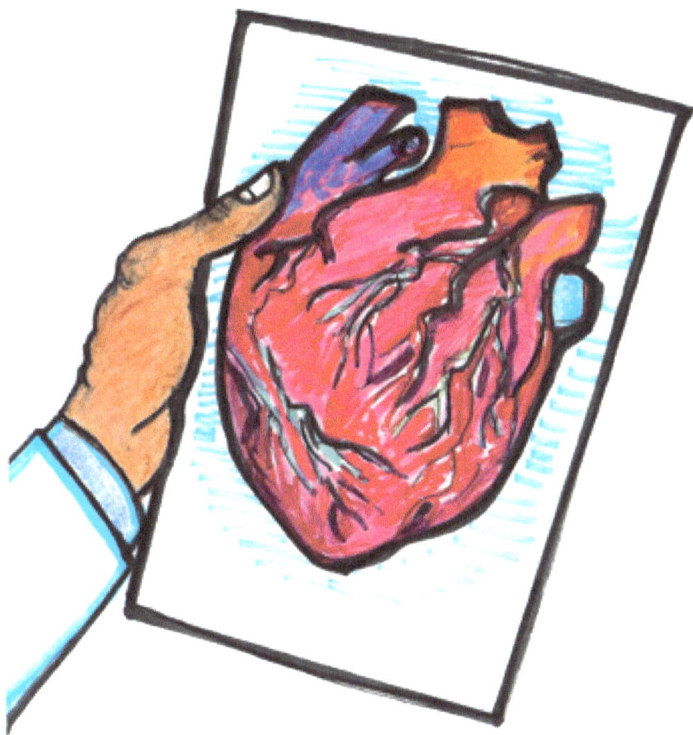

To prevent this, we recommend that you cut
out foods and drinks high in sugar.

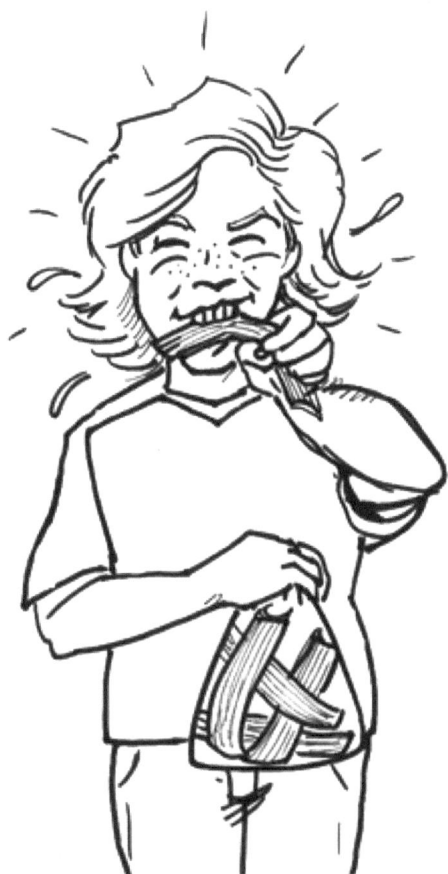

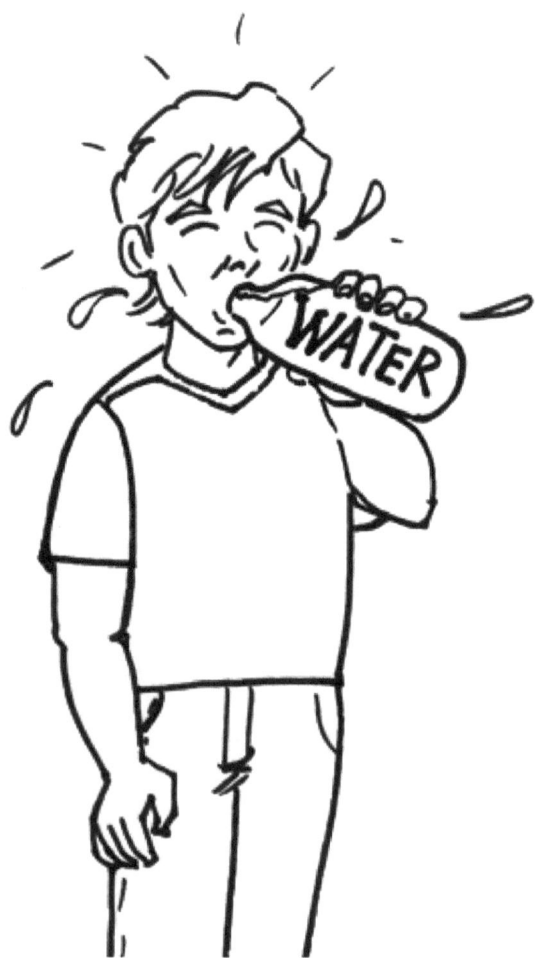

Drink plenty of water.

Drink low fat milk and a small
amount of juice. Eat plenty of fruits
and vegetables.

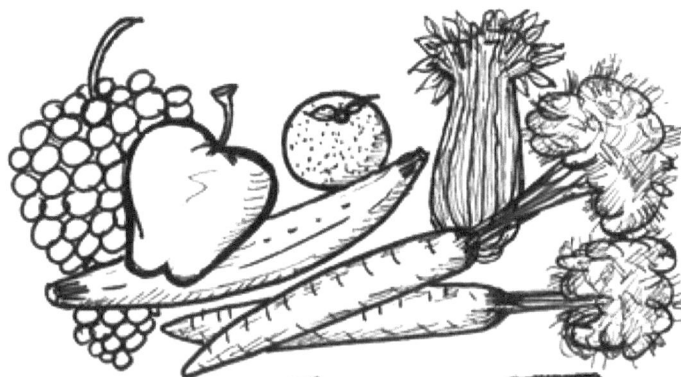

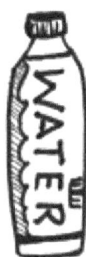

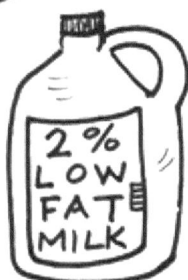

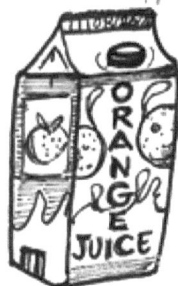

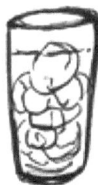

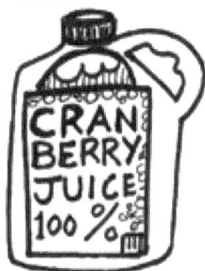

Doing this will lower your risk of obesity, diabetes and heart disease.....

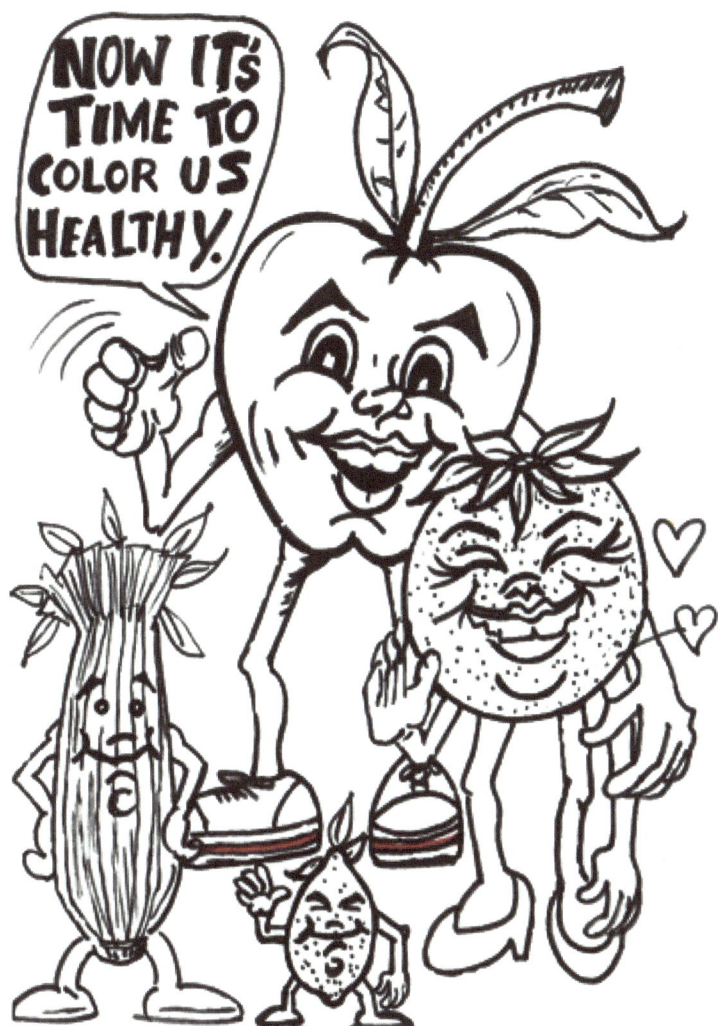

This will lead to a healthier life and your sugar won't be too sweet anymore.

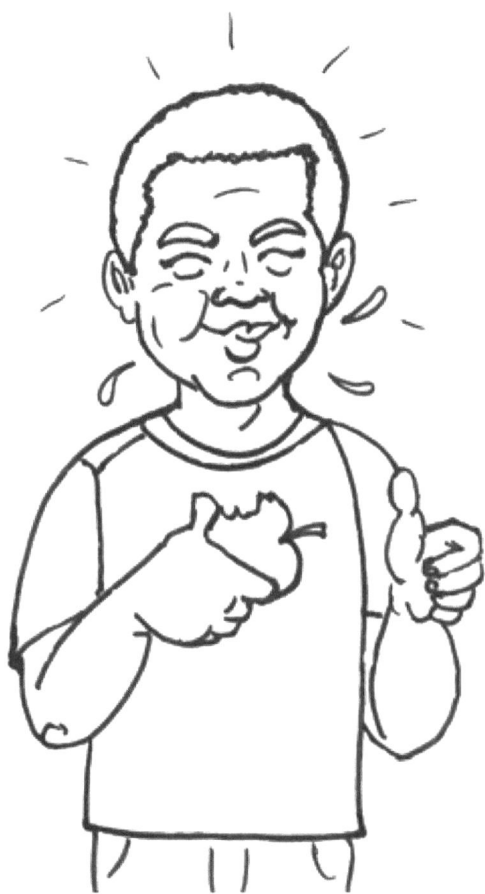

www.ingramcontent.com/pod-product-compliance
Lightning Source LLC
Chambersburg PA
CBHW041215270326
41930CB00001B/34